I0479405

The Frailty Fighter

A Complete Exercise Program for Aging Adults

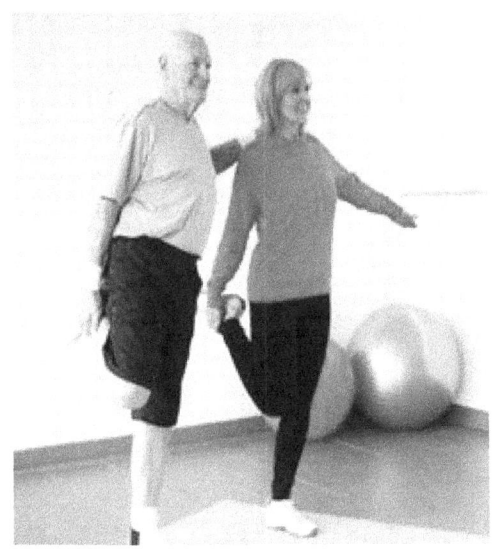

Barbara C. Drake

Table of Content

Introduction

Aging is a natural and inevitable process, but it can be accompanied by challenges and limitations, particularly for those who suffer from frailty syndrome. Frailty syndrome is a condition characterized by decreased strength, balance, and mobility, often leading to falls, hospitalizations, and reduced independence. While frailty syndrome is a common occurrence in aging adults, it is not an unavoidable fate.

Exercise has been shown to be a powerful tool in preventing and managing frailty syndrome. Physical activity can improve muscle strength, balance, cardiovascular function, and cognitive function, leading to increased overall health and well-being. However, for many aging adults, getting started with an exercise program can be intimidating or overwhelming, leading to a lack of motivation and follow-through.

"The Frailty Fighter: A Complete Exercise Program for Aging Adults" is designed to empower aging adults to combat frailty syndrome and maintain their independence through exercise. This comprehensive guide provides a step-by-step exercise program tailored to the specific needs and abilities of aging adults. It covers a wide range of exercises, including strength training, cardiovascular exercise, flexibility, and mobility exercises, as well as special considerations for those with health conditions such as arthritis and osteoporosis.

"The Frailty Fighter" also offers guidance on how to incorporate physical activity into daily routines, set realistic goals, and track progress. It also covers the connection between exercise and mental health, as well as the role of nutrition and hydration in exercise. Whether you are an exercise novice or an experienced athlete, "The Frailty Fighter" offers practical tips and expert advice to help you stay strong and independent as you age.

In this book, we hope to inspire and guide you on your journey to improved health and fitness, and ultimately a more fulfilling life.

Understanding Frailty Syndrome

Frailty syndrome is a condition that affects many aging adults and is characterized by a decline in physical function, strength, and resilience. It is not a single disease, but rather a combination of factors that include chronic health conditions, physical inactivity, poor nutrition, and social isolation.

Frailty is often seen in older adults who have experienced prolonged illnesses or hospitalizations, or who have lost significant amounts of muscle mass due to inactivity or malnutrition. It can lead to increased vulnerability to stressors such as infections, falls, and injuries, which can result in hospitalizations or even death.

There are several common signs and symptoms of frailty syndrome, including decreased muscle mass and strength, poor balance and gait, fatigue, unintentional weight loss, and decreased physical activity. While frailty syndrome is most often associated with aging, it can also affect younger individuals who have experienced prolonged illnesses or inactivity.

It is important to note that frailty syndrome is not a normal part of aging, and can be prevented or managed with lifestyle interventions such as regular physical activity, good nutrition, and social engagement. Identifying and treating frailty early on can also help to improve overall health and quality of life for those affected by the condition.or inactivity.

It is important to note that frailty syndrome is not a normal part of aging, and can be prevented or managed with lifestyle interventions such as regular physical activity, good nutrition, and social engagement. Identifying and treating frailty early on can also help to improve overall health and quality of life for those affected by the condition.

Frailty syndrome can be diagnosed using several different tools and assessments, including the Fried frailty phenotype criteria and the Clinical Frailty Scale. These assessments evaluate various aspects of physical function, such as grip strength, gait speed, and exhaustion, and can help healthcare professionals determine the severity of frailty and the appropriate interventions to address it.

In addition to lifestyle interventions, there are also medical interventions that can be used to manage frailty syndrome. For example, medications may be prescribed to manage underlying health conditions such as hypertension or diabetes, or to improve bone health in those with osteoporosis. Physical therapy and rehabilitation can also be beneficial for improving mobility and balance.

While frailty syndrome can be a challenging condition to manage, there is hope for those affected by it. With the right interventions, including regular exercise and good nutrition, it is possible to improve physical function and overall health. Additionally, social engagement and support can be beneficial for improving mental health and reducing the risk of social isolation, which is a common issue for those with frailty syndrome.

If you or a loved one is experiencing symptoms of frailty syndrome, it is important to speak with a healthcare professional to determine the best course of action. With the right interventions and support, it is possible to improve quality of life and maintain independence for as long as possible.

Why Exercise Is Key to Combating Frailty Syndrome

Exercise is one of the most important interventions for preventing and managing frailty syndrome. Regular physical activity has been shown to improve muscle strength, balance, cardiovascular function, and cognitive function, all of which are important for maintaining independence and reducing the risk of falls and hospitalizations.

Strength training, in particular, is an important component of any exercise program for those with frailty syndrome. This type of exercise helps to build and maintain muscle mass and strength, which can decrease the risk of falls and improve overall physical function. Resistance exercises, such as using weights or resistance bands, have been shown to be effective in improving muscle strength in older adults.

In addition to strength training, cardiovascular exercise is also important for improving overall health and reducing the risk of chronic health conditions such as heart disease and diabetes. Aerobic exercises, such as walking, swimming, or cycling, can also help to improve cardiovascular function and reduce the risk of falls.

Flexibility and mobility exercises, such as stretching and balance exercises, are also important for those with frailty syndrome. These types of exercises can improve range of motion, reduce stiffness and pain, and improve balance and coordination, all of which can help to reduce the risk of falls and improve overall physical function.

It is important to note that exercise should be tailored to the specific needs and abilities of each individual with frailty syndrome. This may involve working with a healthcare professional or certified exercise specialist to design a program that is safe and effective. Additionally, it is important to start slowly and gradually increase the intensity and duration of exercise over time.

It is also important to note that exercise not only benefits physical health, but also mental health. Exercise has been shown to improve mood, reduce stress and anxiety, and improve cognitive function, which can all be important for maintaining overall well-being in older adults.

Furthermore, exercise can also help to combat social isolation, which is a common issue for those with frailty syndrome. Participating in group exercise classes or other physical activities can provide opportunities for social interaction and support, which can be beneficial for mental health and overall quality of life.

In addition to the physical and mental health benefits of exercise, there are also economic benefits to preventing and managing frailty syndrome through exercise. Frailty syndrome can result in increased healthcare costs, including hospitalizations and long-term care, which can be a significant burden on individuals and the healthcare system as a whole. By promoting exercise and other lifestyle interventions for preventing and managing frailty syndrome, healthcare costs can be reduced and overall health outcomes can be improved.

In summary, exercise is a key intervention for preventing and managing frailty syndrome. It can improve muscle strength, balance, cardiovascular function, cognitive function, mental health, and social interaction, all of which are important for maintaining independence and overall well-being. By incorporating exercise into daily routines and promoting physical activity for older adults, we can work to prevent and manage frailty syndrome and improve overall health outcomes for individuals and society as a whole.

Setting Realistic Goals

When it comes to exercise for those with frailty syndrome, setting realistic goals is essential for success. It is important to remember that exercise should be tailored to each individual's abilities and needs, and that progress may be slower than expected due to the limitations imposed by frailty syndrome.

One effective approach to goal setting is to use the SMART framework. SMART stands for Specific, Measurable, Attainable, Relevant, and Time-bound. Here's what each of these components means:

- Specific: Set clear and specific goals. For example, "I will walk for 10 minutes every day" is more specific than "I will exercise more."
- Measurable: Set goals that can be tracked and measured. For example, "I will increase my walking speed by 10% within the next month" is more measurable than "I will walk more."
- Attainable: Set goals that are challenging but realistic. It is important to consider individual abilities and limitations when setting goals. For example, "I will walk for 10 minutes every day" may be attainable for some individuals, while others may need to start with shorter walks.
- Relevant: Set goals that are relevant to overall health and well-being. For example, goals that target muscle strength, balance, and cardiovascular

health are all relevant for those with frailty syndrome.

- Time-bound: Set goals with a specific timeline. For example, "I will walk for 10 minutes every day for the next month" is more time-bound than "I will walk more."

By setting SMART goals, individuals with frailty syndrome can track their progress and feel a sense of accomplishment as they reach their goals. It is important to remember that progress may be slow, and setbacks may occur, but with persistence and determination, individuals can achieve their goals and improve their overall health and well-being.

In addition to using the SMART framework, it is also important to consider other factors when setting exercise goals for those with frailty syndrome. These may include:

- Starting with small goals: It may be helpful to start with small goals, such as walking for 5-10 minutes a day, and gradually increase the intensity and duration of exercise over time.
- Including variety: Incorporating a variety of exercises, such as resistance training, balance exercises, and aerobic activity, can help to target multiple aspects of physical function and prevent boredom.
- Considering safety: Safety should always be a top priority when exercising with frailty syndrome. It may be necessary to modify exercises or use assistive devices to ensure safety.
- Listening to the body: It is important to pay attention to how the body feels

during and after exercise. If an exercise causes pain or discomfort, it may be necessary to adjust or modify the exercise.

- Celebrating progress: Celebrating even small progress can help to maintain motivation and momentum. Whether it's reaching a new walking distance or lifting a heavier weight, acknowledging and celebrating progress can help to build confidence and self-esteem.

Ultimately, the key to successful goal setting for exercise with frailty syndrome is to keep goals realistic, flexible, and tailored to individual needs and abilities. With patience, persistence, and support from healthcare professionals and loved ones, individuals with frailty syndrome can achieve their exercise goals and improve their overall health and well-being.

Chapter 1

Preparing for Exercise

Before beginning any exercise program, it is important to prepare both physically and mentally. This is especially true for individuals with frailty syndrome, who may have unique physical limitations and challenges. Here are some tips for preparing for exercise:

1. Consult with a healthcare professional: It is important to consult with a healthcare professional, such as a doctor or physical therapist, before beginning any exercise program. This is especially important for individuals with frailty syndrome, who may have

underlying health conditions that need to be considered.

2. Set realistic goals: Setting realistic goals can help to maintain motivation and prevent frustration. It is important to consider individual abilities and limitations when setting goals.

3. Choose appropriate exercises: Exercises should be tailored to individual needs and abilities. Resistance training, balance exercises, and cardiovascular exercise can all be beneficial for those with frailty syndrome.

4. Warm-up and cool down: A proper warm-up and cool down can help to prevent injury and improve performance. A warm-up may include light aerobic exercise and stretching,

while a cool down may include
stretching and gentle movement.

5. Consider assistive devices: Assistive
   devices, such as canes or walkers, may
   be necessary to ensure safety and
   improve mobility.

6. Wear appropriate clothing and
   footwear: Clothing and footwear
   should be comfortable, breathable, and
   supportive.

By preparing both physically and mentally
before beginning an exercise program,
individuals with frailty syndrome can
increase their chances of success and reduce
the risk of injury. It is important to listen to
the body and adjust exercises as needed, and
to seek support and guidance from healthcare
professionals and loved ones.

Safety Precautions

Safety is a top priority when it comes to exercise, particularly for individuals with frailty syndrome. Here are some safety precautions to consider before starting an exercise program:

1. Consult with a healthcare professional: As mentioned before, it is important to consult with a healthcare professional before beginning any exercise program. This can help to identify any potential risks or limitations and ensure that exercises are safe and appropriate.

2. Start slow and progress gradually: Starting with low-intensity exercises and gradually increasing intensity and duration can help to prevent injury and improve overall fitness. Pushing too

hard too soon can lead to injury or burnout.

3. Use assistive devices: Assistive devices, such as canes or walkers, can improve safety and balance during exercise. They should be used as needed and properly adjusted to ensure proper alignment and stability.

4. Choose safe environments: Exercise should be done in safe and appropriate environments, such as a gym or physical therapy clinic, with appropriate equipment and supervision. Avoid exercising in hazardous or unstable environments, such as uneven terrain or dimly lit areas.

5. Stay hydrated: Staying hydrated is important for overall health and can help to prevent dizziness and fatigue during exercise.

6. Listen to the body: Pay attention to any pain or discomfort during exercise and

adjust as needed. Pushing through pain or discomfort can lead to injury.

7. Take breaks when needed: Rest breaks can help to prevent fatigue and improve overall performance. Take breaks as needed and don't push past your limits.

8. Monitor vital signs: Individuals with frailty syndrome may have underlying health conditions that need to be monitored during exercise. This may include monitoring heart rate, blood pressure, and oxygen saturation levels. If these levels exceed safe ranges, it may be necessary to adjust exercise intensity or take a break.

9. Avoid high-risk exercises: Some exercises may be too high-risk for individuals with frailty syndrome, such as high-impact exercises or exercises that require sudden changes in direction. These exercises should be

avoided or modified to reduce risk of injury.

10. Consider a supervised exercise program: A supervised exercise program, such as a physical therapy program, can provide additional guidance and support in a safe and monitored environment. This can be particularly beneficial for individuals with frailty syndrome who may have additional limitations or health concerns.

11. Keep emergency information on hand: It is important to keep emergency information, such as contact information for healthcare professionals and emergency services, on hand during exercise. This can help to ensure quick access to help in the event of an emergency.

By taking these additional safety precautions, individuals with frailty syndrome can further minimize the risk of injury and maximize the benefits of exercise. It is important to be proactive in ensuring safety during exercise, and to seek guidance and support from healthcare professionals and loved ones as needed.

Finding the Right Equipment

Finding the right equipment is an important part of ensuring safety and effectiveness during exercise, particularly for individuals with frailty syndrome. Here are some considerations to keep in mind when selecting equipment:

1. Stability and support: Equipment should provide stability and support during exercise, particularly for exercises that require balance or weight-bearing. This may include using

a stability ball or resistance bands for added support.

2. Adjustability: Equipment should be adjustable to ensure proper alignment and accommodate individual needs and limitations. This may include adjusting the height or angle of equipment, or using custom-made equipment for specific needs.

3. Low-impact options: Low-impact exercise equipment, such as elliptical machines or stationary bikes, can be beneficial for individuals with frailty syndrome who may have joint pain or limited mobility.

4. Assistive devices: Assistive devices, such as canes or walkers, can also be used as exercise equipment to provide additional support and stability during exercise.

5. Comfort and safety: Equipment should be comfortable and safe to use, with

appropriate padding or grips to reduce risk of injury or discomfort.

6. Cost: Equipment can range in cost, so it is important to consider individual budgets when selecting equipment. It may also be possible to find low-cost or second-hand equipment options.

7. Accessibility: Equipment should be accessible and easy to use, particularly for individuals with limited mobility or other disabilities.

8. User-friendly: The equipment should be easy to assemble and use. Individuals with frailty syndrome may have limited mobility or may require assistance to use equipment. Therefore, the equipment should be user-friendly and easy to operate with clear instructions.

9. Space requirements: The amount of space required for equipment should also be considered. Individuals with

limited space may opt for equipment that can be easily stored or folded away when not in use.

10.   Durability: The equipment should be durable and long-lasting to ensure that it can withstand repeated use. This can help to minimize the need for frequent repairs or replacements, which can be costly and inconvenient.

11.   Personal preference: Ultimately, personal preference should also be considered when selecting equipment. Individuals should select equipment that they enjoy using and that fits their interests and needs.

Finding the right exercise equipment can be a daunting task, particularly for individuals with frailty syndrome. However, with careful consideration of the above factors, individuals can select equipment that is safe, effective, and appropriate for their individual needs and limitations. It is important to seek guidance and support from healthcare professionals and loved ones as needed when selecting and using exercise equipment.

Setting Up Your Space

Creating a safe and comfortable space for exercise is an important part of ensuring success and minimizing risk of injury for individuals with frailty syndrome. Here are some considerations to keep in mind when setting up a space for exercise:

1. Clear the space: Clear the space of any objects or obstacles that could pose a tripping hazard. This may include rugs, furniture, or clutter.
2. Adequate lighting: The space should be well-lit to ensure visibility during exercise. Natural light is preferable, but

if not available, artificial lighting can be used.

3. Ventilation: The space should have adequate ventilation to ensure comfort during exercise. This may include opening windows or using a fan.

4. Flooring: The flooring should be appropriate for exercise, with sufficient cushioning to reduce impact on joints. Hardwood, rubber or foam flooring can be good options.

5. Adequate space: The space should have adequate space for exercise, with enough room to move freely and safely.

6. Storage: Storage should be provided for equipment to ensure that it is organized and easily accessible. This may include shelves, cabinets, or storage bins.

7. Personal touches: Adding personal touches, such as music or motivational posters, can help to create a

comfortable and motivating environment for exercise.

8. Accessibility: The space should also be accessible for individuals with limited mobility or assistive devices, such as wheelchairs or walkers. This may include ramps, grab bars, or other modifications to ensure that the space is fully accessible for all users.

9. Temperature control: The temperature of the space should also be considered, with a comfortable temperature range that allows for safe and comfortable exercise.

10. Privacy: Some individuals may prefer a private space for exercise, free from distractions or interruptions. This can be achieved by selecting a quiet and secluded location or using privacy screens.

11. Safety equipment: It is also important to have safety equipment on

hand in case of emergencies, such as a first aid kit or phone for emergency services.

By taking these additional considerations into account, individuals with frailty syndrome can further enhance the safety and comfort of their exercise space, ensuring a successful and enjoyable exercise experience. It is important to consult with healthcare professionals and loved ones to identify any additional needs or modifications that may be necessary to optimize the exercise space for individual needs and preferences.

Stretching and Warming Up

Stretching and warming up are crucial steps in preparing the body for exercise, particularly for individuals with frailty syndrome. Here are some considerations to keep in mind when stretching and warming up:

1. Start slow: Begin with gentle movements to gradually increase heart rate and body temperature. This may include walking or gentle stretches.
2. Focus on major muscle groups: Focus on stretching major muscle groups, such as the quadriceps, hamstrings, and back muscles.
3. Hold stretches: Hold stretches for at least 30 seconds to allow for adequate muscle elongation and flexibility.
4. Use slow and controlled movements: Use slow and controlled movements to minimize the risk of injury and

maximize the effectiveness of the stretch.

5. Avoid bouncing: Avoid bouncing or jerking movements, which can lead to injury.

6. Breathe deeply: Focus on deep breathing during stretching to help promote relaxation and reduce stress.

7. Use props: Props, such as yoga blocks or resistance bands, can be used to enhance the effectiveness of stretches.

8. Consider dynamic stretching: Dynamic stretching involves moving through a range of motion rather than holding a static stretch. This type of stretching can be particularly beneficial for individuals with frailty syndrome, as it can help to improve mobility and flexibility.

9. Gradually increase intensity: Gradually increase the intensity of warm-up exercises to further prepare the body

for exercise. This may include increasing the speed or resistance of a cardio machine or adding weight to strength training exercises.

10. Listen to your body: Pay attention to your body during stretching and warming up. If any stretches or movements feel uncomfortable or painful, modify or skip them as needed.

11. Warm up before strength training: Prior to strength training, it is important to perform a specific warm-up for the muscles being targeted. This may include performing a few repetitions of the exercise with lighter weights or resistance.

By incorporating these additional considerations into their stretching and warming up routine, individuals with frailty syndrome can further optimize their exercise experience and minimize the risk of injury. It is important to seek guidance and support from healthcare professionals and loved ones as needed when designing a stretching and warming up routine that is safe and effective for individual needs and preferences.

Chapter 2

Building Strength and Balance

Building strength and balance are essential components of a successful exercise program for individuals with frailty syndrome. Here are some considerations to keep in mind when building strength and balance:

1. Start with low resistance: Begin with low resistance or bodyweight exercises to gradually build strength and reduce the risk of injury. This may include exercises such as squats, lunges, and push-ups.

2. Focus on major muscle groups: Focus on strengthening major muscle groups, such as the legs, hips, back, and chest,

to improve overall strength and balance.

3. Use proper form: Use proper form when performing exercises to maximize effectiveness and minimize the risk of injury. This may include maintaining a neutral spine, engaging core muscles, and keeping the knees in line with the toes during lower body exercises.

4. Incorporate balance exercises: Incorporate balance exercises, such as standing on one leg or practicing tai chi, to improve balance and reduce the risk of falls.

5. Gradually increase resistance: Gradually increase the resistance or weight used in exercises as strength and endurance improve. This can help

to continually challenge the body and promote further improvements in strength and balance.

6. Use safety equipment: Use safety equipment, such as a chair or stability ball, to provide additional support and safety during exercises.

7. Consider working with a professional: Consider working with a fitness professional or physical therapist to develop a safe and effective strength and balance program that is tailored to individual needs and preferences.

Resistance Band Exercises

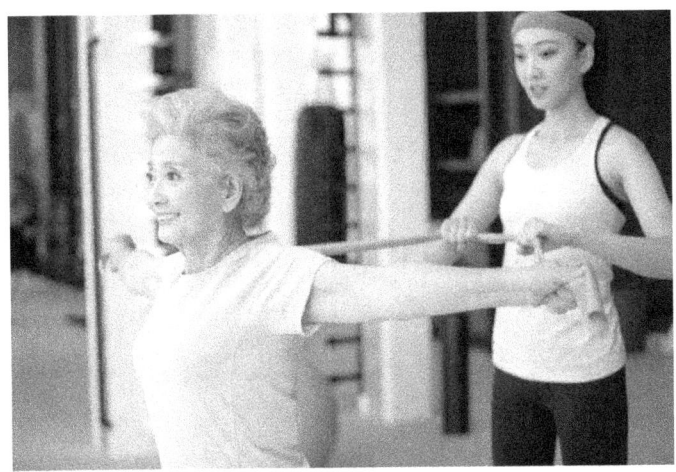

Resistance bands are a versatile and convenient tool for individuals with frailty syndrome to incorporate into their exercise routine. Here are some resistance band exercises to consider:

1. Seated row: Sit on the floor with your legs extended in front of you and loop the resistance band around your feet. Grasp the handles and pull them towards your body, squeezing your

shoulder blades together. Release and repeat.

2. Leg press: Loop the resistance band around a sturdy object, such as a table leg or bedpost. Place one foot in the loop and step back until there is tension in the band. Bend the knee of the foot in the loop to press the band down towards the ground. Release and repeat on the other side.

3. Chest press: Securely attach the resistance band to a stable object at chest height. Stand facing away from the object and grasp the handles. Push the handles forward, keeping the elbows close to the body. Release and repeat.

4. Bicep curl: Stand on the center of the resistance band with feet shoulder-width apart. Grasp the handles and curl them towards your shoulders,

keeping the elbows close to the body.
Release and repeat.

5. Lateral raise: Stand on the center of the
   resistance band with feet
   shoulder-width apart. Grasp the handles
   and lift your arms out to the side,
   keeping them straight. Release and
   repeat.

Resistance band exercises can provide
individuals with frailty syndrome with an
effective way to build strength, improve
balance, and increase overall physical
function. Resistance bands come in a variety
of shapes, sizes, and resistance levels,
allowing for a customized workout
experience that can be adjusted as strength
and ability improve.

One of the many benefits of resistance band
exercises is their versatility. They can be
easily adapted to fit an individual's specific
needs and preferences, and can be used in a

variety of settings. For example, resistance band exercises can be performed while seated, standing, or lying down, making them accessible to individuals with a range of mobility levels.

In addition to being versatile, resistance band exercises can also help to improve joint stability and mobility. By providing controlled resistance, resistance bands can help to improve muscle and joint activation, which can lead to improved mobility and reduced joint pain. This is particularly beneficial for individuals with frailty syndrome, who may be experiencing joint pain or stiffness as a result of age or injury.

When incorporating resistance band exercises into an exercise routine, it is important to prioritize safety and proper technique. This may include using proper form, selecting the appropriate resistance level, and using safety equipment such as a chair or stability ball as needed.

Overall, resistance band exercises can be an effective and convenient way for individuals with frailty syndrome to improve their strength, balance, and overall physical function. It is important to consult with healthcare professionals and loved ones to identify any individual needs or modifications that may be necessary for resistance band exercises, such as modifications for joint pain or limited mobility.

Bodyweight Exercises

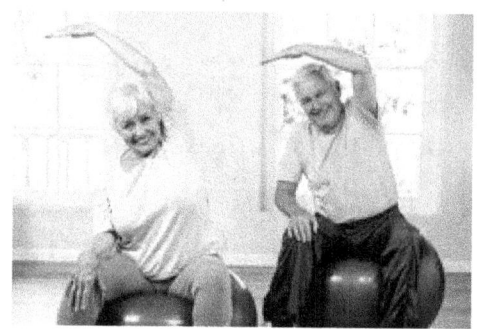

Bodyweight exercises are a simple and effective way for individuals with frailty syndrome to build strength, improve balance, and increase overall physical function. Here are some bodyweight exercises to consider:

1. Sit to stand: Sit in a sturdy chair with feet flat on the ground. Stand up from the chair using leg strength, then slowly lower back down to a seated position. Repeat.
2. Wall push-ups: Stand facing a wall with feet shoulder-width apart. Place hands on the wall at shoulder height

and perform push-ups by bending elbows and lowering body towards the wall. Push back up to starting position and repeat.

3. Single-leg balance: Stand near a sturdy surface for support, such as a chair or wall. Lift one foot off the ground and balance on the other foot for a few seconds. Lower and repeat on the other side.

4. Plank: Begin on hands and knees with hands shoulder-width apart. Extend legs back, keeping toes on the ground, and engage core muscles to hold a straight line from head to heels. Hold for 10-30 seconds, then release.

5. Lunges: Stand with feet shoulder-width apart and step forward with one foot. Lower back knee towards the ground, keeping front knee at a 90-degree angle. Push back up to starting position and repeat on the other side.

When incorporating bodyweight exercises into an exercise routine, it is important to prioritize safety and proper technique. This may include using proper form, selecting the appropriate exercise intensity, and using safety equipment such as a chair or stability ball as needed. It is also important to gradually increase the number of repetitions or sets over time to avoid overexertion or injury.

Bodyweight exercises can be a great way for individuals with frailty syndrome to improve their strength and balance, but it is important to remember that every individual's needs and abilities are different. It is recommended to consult with healthcare professionals and loved ones to determine the appropriate exercises and modifications for an individual's specific needs and abilities.

In addition to their physical benefits, bodyweight exercises can also have positive impacts on mental health and wellbeing. Exercise has been shown to improve mood, reduce stress and anxiety, and increase overall feelings of wellbeing. By incorporating bodyweight exercises into a regular exercise routine, individuals with frailty syndrome can experience not only physical benefits, but also emotional and mental benefits.

Bodyweight exercises can be easily modified to accommodate individual needs and abilities, such as by adjusting the intensity or performing exercises seated instead of standing. Additionally, bodyweight exercises can be performed anywhere without the need for equipment, making them a convenient option for at-home workouts. It is important to seek guidance and support from healthcare professionals and loved ones as needed when incorporating bodyweight exercises into an exercise routine.

Weight Training

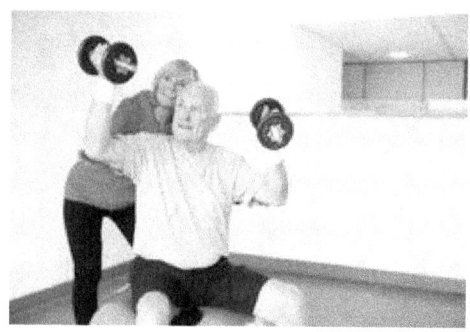

Weight training, also known as resistance training or strength training, involves using weights or resistance to improve muscular strength and endurance. It can be a beneficial exercise for individuals with frailty syndrome, as it can help to maintain and increase muscle mass, improve bone density, and enhance overall physical function.

Here are some weight training exercises to consider:

1. Squats: Hold a weight or use a resistance band and stand with feet shoulder-width apart. Lower into a squat, keeping weight in heels and knees aligned with toes. Push back up to starting position and repeat.

2. Chest press: Lie on a bench or the floor and hold a weight in each hand. With arms extended, lower weights towards chest, then push back up to starting position and repeat.

3. Bicep curls: Stand with feet shoulder-width apart and hold a weight in each hand. With palms facing up, bend elbows and bring weights towards shoulders. Lower back down to starting position and repeat.

4. Leg press: Use a leg press machine or resistance band and place feet on platform. Push platform away from body with legs, then slowly lower back down and repeat.

5. Shoulder press: Sit or stand with feet shoulder-width apart and hold a weight in each hand. With arms extended, lift weights up towards shoulders, then push up overhead. Lower back down to starting position and repeat.

Weight training exercises can be modified to accommodate individual needs and abilities, such as adjusting the weight or selecting exercises that target specific muscle groups. It is important to seek guidance and support from healthcare professionals and loved ones as needed when incorporating weight training into an exercise routine.

In addition to its physical benefits, weight training can also have positive impacts on mental health and wellbeing. Exercise has been shown to improve mood, reduce stress and anxiety, and increase overall feelings of wellbeing. By incorporating weight training into a regular exercise routine, individuals with frailty syndrome can experience not only physical benefits, but also emotional and mental benefits.

When incorporating weight training into an exercise routine, it is important to start with lighter weights and gradually increase weight and intensity over time. This allows the body to adapt and reduce the risk of injury. It is also important to use proper form and technique when performing exercises to ensure safety and effectiveness.

In addition to traditional weight training exercises, individuals with frailty syndrome may also benefit from using resistance bands or bodyweight exercises as a form of strength training. These exercises can be performed with little to no equipment and can be modified to suit individual needs and abilities.

Resistance bands are elastic bands that can be used to provide resistance during exercise. They are portable and easy to use, making them a convenient option for individuals who may not have access to a gym or weight equipment. Resistance bands can be used for a variety of exercises, such as bicep curls, chest presses, and leg extensions.

Bodyweight exercises involve using one's own body weight as resistance during exercise. Examples include push-ups, squats, and lunges. Bodyweight exercises can be modified to accommodate individual abilities and can be performed at home or in a gym setting.

Incorporating weight training exercises, resistance band exercises, and bodyweight exercises into an exercise routine can help to improve strength, balance, and overall physical function for individuals with frailty syndrome. It is important to consult with a

healthcare professional before beginning a
new exercise routine and to seek guidance
and support as needed.

Core Strengthening

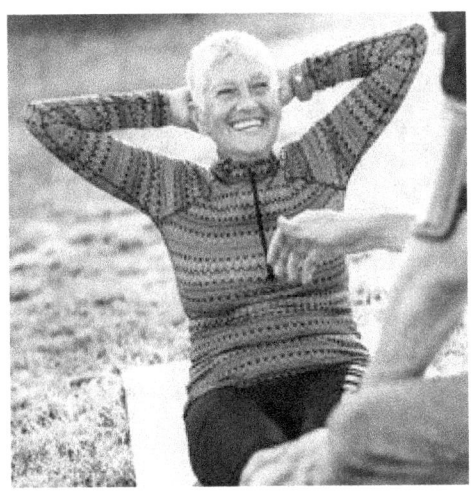

Core strengthening exercises are an important
aspect of any exercise routine, especially for
individuals with frailty syndrome. The core
muscles include the abdominals, back
muscles, and muscles around the hips and
pelvis. These muscles are important for
maintaining balance and stability, as well as

for performing everyday activities such as bending, lifting, and reaching.

There are many exercises that can help to strengthen the core muscles, including:

1. Plank: The plank is a simple but effective exercise that involves holding a straight, neutral spine position for a period of time. To perform a plank, start in a push-up position with your elbows on the ground and your forearms flat on the floor. Keep your body in a straight line from head to heels, engaging your core muscles throughout the exercise.

2. Bridges: Bridges target the muscles in the hips, buttocks, and lower back. To perform a bridge, lie on your back with your knees bent and feet flat on the ground. Lift your hips off the ground, squeezing your glutes and engaging your core muscles as you lift.

3. Bird dog: The bird dog exercise targets the muscles in the back and core. To perform the bird dog, start on your hands and knees with your hands directly under your shoulders and your knees directly under your hips. Extend one arm and the opposite leg out straight, keeping your core muscles engaged and your spine in a neutral position. Return to the starting position and repeat on the other side.

4. Russian twist: The Russian twist targets the obliques, the muscles on the sides of the abdomen. To perform a Russian twist, sit on the ground with your knees bent and your feet flat on the ground. Lean back slightly, keeping your back straight, and lift your feet off the ground. Twist your torso to the right, then to the left, while holding a weight or medicine ball in your hands.

5. Side plank: The side plank targets the muscles on the sides of the body, including the obliques and the hips. To perform a side plank, lie on your side with your elbow directly under your shoulder and your legs straight. Lift your hips off the ground, keeping your body in a straight line from head to heels. Hold for a period of time, then switch sides.

6. Dead bug: The dead bug exercise targets the deep core muscles and helps to improve coordination and stability. To perform a dead bug, lie on your back with your arms extended towards the ceiling and your knees bent at a 90-degree angle. Slowly lower one arm and the opposite leg towards the ground, keeping your core engaged and your lower back flat on the ground. Return to the starting position and repeat on the other side.

Incorporating a variety of core strengthening exercises into an exercise routine can help to improve overall physical function and reduce the risk of falls and injuries for individuals with frailty syndrome. As with any exercise routine, it is important to consult with a healthcare professional before beginning and to seek guidance and support as needed.

Chapter 3

Cardiovascular Exercise

In addition to building strength and balance, cardiovascular exercise is an essential component of a well-rounded exercise program for individuals with frailty syndrome. Regular cardiovascular exercise can improve heart health, reduce the risk of chronic diseases, and enhance overall physical function.

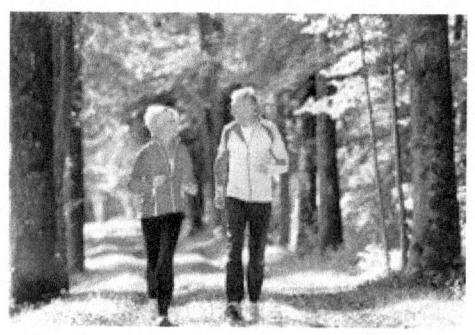

1. Walking: Walking is a low-impact form of cardiovascular exercise that can be easily incorporated into daily routines. Aim for at least 30 minutes of walking each day, or break it up into shorter sessions throughout the day.

2. Cycling: Cycling is another low-impact form of cardiovascular exercise that can be done indoors or outdoors. Stationary bikes are a great option for individuals with limited mobility or balance issues.

3. Swimming: Swimming is a low-impact form of cardiovascular exercise that is gentle on the joints and can be a great option for individuals with mobility issues. Many community centers and gyms offer swim classes for seniors.

4. Dancing: Dancing is a fun way to get moving and improve cardiovascular health. Many community centers and dance studios offer classes specifically for seniors.

5. Chair aerobics: Chair aerobics are a low-impact form of cardiovascular exercise that can be done from a seated position. They are a great option for individuals with limited mobility or balance issues.

6. treadmill or elliptical: A treadmill or elliptical machine can be a great option for individuals who prefer to exercise indoors. These machines provide a low-impact cardiovascular workout that can be adjusted to individual fitness levels.

7. Tai chi: Tai chi is a gentle form of exercise that combines slow, flowing movements with deep breathing and relaxation techniques. It can help improve balance, flexibility, and cardiovascular health.

8. Yoga: Yoga is a gentle form of exercise that can improve flexibility, balance, and overall physical function. It can be done in a group setting or at home using online videos or DVDs.

When starting a cardiovascular exercise program, it is important to choose activities that you enjoy and that are appropriate for your fitness level. Gradually increase the intensity and duration of your workouts, but listen to your body and rest when needed. Be sure to warm up before each session and cool down afterwards to prevent injury.

Remember, any amount of cardiovascular exercise is better than none. Even a few minutes of walking or dancing can provide health benefits. Consistency is key, so try to make exercise a regular part of your routine. With time and effort, you can improve your cardiovascular health and overall physical function.

It is important to start slow and gradually increase the intensity and duration of cardiovascular exercise. Aim for at least 150 minutes of moderate-intensity cardiovascular exercise per week, or 75 minutes of vigorous-intensity cardiovascular exercise per week, spread out over at least three days.

Always consult with a healthcare professional before starting a new exercise program, especially if you have a chronic condition or are taking medications that may affect your heart rate or blood pressure.

Walking

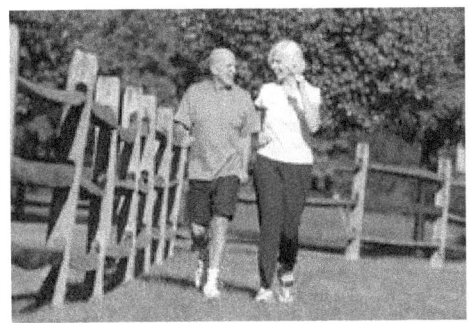

Walking is a simple and low-impact form of cardiovascular exercise that is suitable for individuals with frailty syndrome. It can be done outdoors or indoors on a treadmill, and can easily be incorporated into daily routines.

One of the benefits of walking is that it can be done at any time of day, for any duration of time. Even a short walk around the block can provide health benefits such as improved cardiovascular health, increased muscle strength and endurance, and better mental health.

To start a walking program, begin with short walks of 5-10 minutes at a comfortable pace. Gradually increase the duration and intensity of your walks over time. Aim for at least 30 minutes of walking per day, or break it up into two or three shorter sessions throughout the day.

When walking outdoors, wear comfortable and supportive shoes, dress appropriately for the weather, and stay hydrated. It's also important to be aware of your surroundings and to walk on flat, even surfaces to reduce the risk of falls.

If walking outdoors is not an option, consider using a treadmill or walking indoors at a community center or gym. Many facilities offer walking programs or walking groups for seniors.

Walking is a safe and effective form of exercise that can be tailored to fit your fitness level and personal preferences. It can also be modified to accommodate physical limitations or health conditions. For example, individuals with frailty syndrome can start with short, slow walks and gradually increase the duration and intensity of their walks as they build strength and endurance.

In addition to physical health benefits, walking can also have a positive impact on mental health. Walking can reduce stress and anxiety, improve mood, and boost cognitive function. Walking outdoors in nature can also provide a sense of relaxation and connection with the natural world.

To keep your walking routine interesting, consider varying your route or exploring new walking paths in your community. You can also listen to music, audiobooks, or podcasts to keep you engaged and motivated. Walking with a friend or in a group can also provide social support and make the experience more enjoyable.

Walking is an excellent way to improve cardiovascular health, increase physical function, and enhance overall well-being. By incorporating walking into your daily routine, you can improve your health and quality of life.

Jogging and Running

jogging and running are high-impact forms of cardiovascular exercise that can provide significant health benefits for individuals with frailty syndrome. However, it is important to approach these activities with caution and to gradually build up intensity to avoid injury.

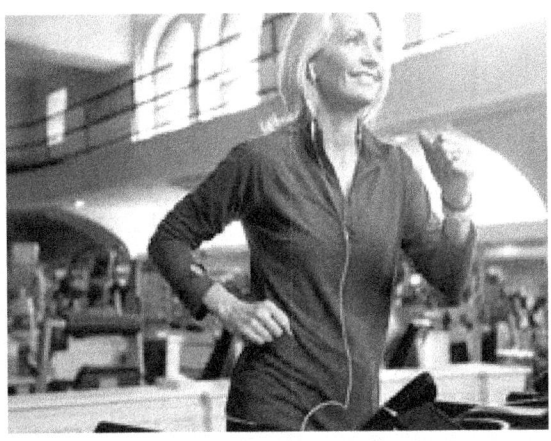

Jogging and running can improve cardiovascular health, increase muscle strength and endurance, and promote weight loss. These activities also have mental health benefits, such as reducing stress and anxiety and improving mood.

Before beginning a jogging or running program, it is important to consult with a healthcare provider to determine if it is safe for you to engage in high-impact exercise.

You should also invest in a pair of supportive and cushioned running shoes to reduce the risk of injury.

To begin a jogging or running program, start with short intervals of jogging or running interspersed with walking. Gradually increase the duration and intensity of the jogging or running intervals and decrease the walking intervals as you build endurance. It is also important to incorporate rest days into your program to allow for recovery.

If you experience pain or discomfort while jogging or running, stop and consult with a healthcare provider. It is also important to listen to your body and modify your program as needed to avoid overexertion or injury.

It is important to note that jogging and running may not be suitable for everyone with frailty syndrome, particularly if there are preexisting health conditions that make high-impact exercise unsafe. In these cases, low-impact cardio exercises like walking or stationary cycling may be more appropriate.

If you do decide to incorporate jogging or running into your exercise routine, it is important to pay attention to proper form to avoid injury. This includes landing on the middle of your foot, keeping your strides short and quick, and keeping your head up and shoulders relaxed.

To make jogging or running more enjoyable, consider varying your route or terrain, running with a friend or group, or listening to music or podcasts. You can also set goals for yourself, such as running a certain distance or completing a 5k race.

As with any exercise program, it is important to start slowly and gradually build up intensity to avoid injury or overexertion. Always listen to your body and modify your program as needed to accommodate physical limitations or health conditions.

Overall, jogging and running can be effective forms of exercise for individuals with frailty syndrome, but it is important to approach these activities with caution and to consult with a healthcare provider before beginning a high-impact exercise program. With proper form and gradual progression, jogging and running can improve physical function, cardiovascular health, and overall well-being.

Cycling

Cycling is another great cardiovascular exercise that can be suitable for individuals with frailty syndrome. Cycling can be done outdoors on a bicycle or indoors on a stationary bike, making it a versatile option for people with different preferences and abilities.

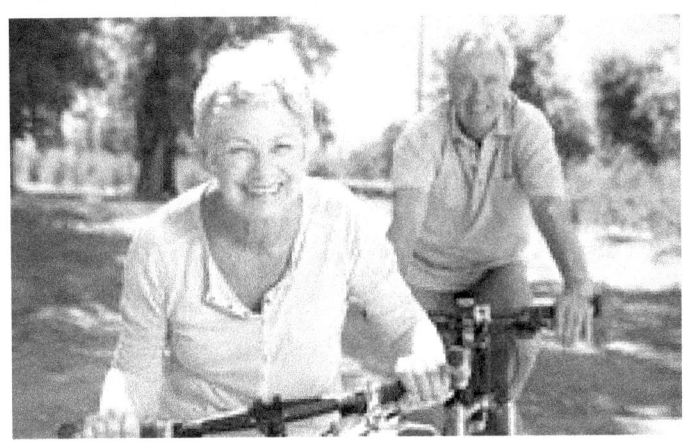

Cycling provides a low-impact workout that is gentle on the joints while still offering a challenging cardiovascular workout. It can improve heart health, lung capacity, and overall endurance. Additionally, cycling can also help to build lower body strength, particularly in the quads, hamstrings, and glutes.

When cycling, it is important to ensure that you have proper equipment, including a well-fitted helmet and comfortable clothing. For outdoor cycling, it is also important to follow traffic laws and ride defensively to stay safe on the road.

Indoor cycling classes are a popular option for those who prefer to exercise in a group setting or who may not feel comfortable cycling outdoors. These classes often incorporate upbeat music and interval training to keep participants engaged and motivated.

As with any exercise program, it is important to start slowly and gradually increase intensity to avoid injury or overexertion. Always listen to your body and modify your program as needed to accommodate physical limitations or health conditions.

Overall, cycling can be an effective and enjoyable form of exercise for individuals with frailty syndrome. Whether done outdoors or indoors, cycling can improve cardiovascular health, build lower body strength, and enhance overall well-being.

Swimming

Swimming is an excellent form of cardiovascular exercise that can be particularly beneficial for individuals with frailty syndrome. The buoyancy of the water can reduce impact on the joints, making it a low-impact option for those who may have limited mobility or joint pain.

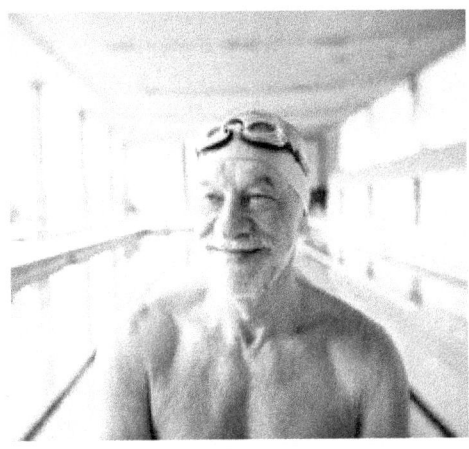

Swimming engages the entire body and can help to improve cardiovascular health, lung capacity, and endurance. It can also help to build strength and flexibility, particularly in the arms, shoulders, and back.

One of the advantages of swimming is that it offers a wide variety of workout options, including lap swimming, water aerobics, and water jogging. Water aerobics classes can provide a fun and social environment for exercise, while water jogging can offer a more challenging workout that is still gentle on the joints.

When swimming, it is important to ensure that you have proper equipment, including a well-fitted swimsuit and goggles. It is also important to take precautions to avoid accidents or injuries, such as swimming with a buddy and using caution when diving or jumping into the pool.

Swimming can be an effective and enjoyable form of exercise for individuals with frailty syndrome. It provides a low-impact workout that can improve cardiovascular health, build strength and flexibility, and enhance overall well-being.

Chair Cardio

Chair cardio is a great option for individuals with frailty syndrome who may have limited mobility or difficulty standing for long periods of time. Chair cardio exercises involve using a chair as a support while performing cardiovascular movements that raise the heart rate and increase circulation.

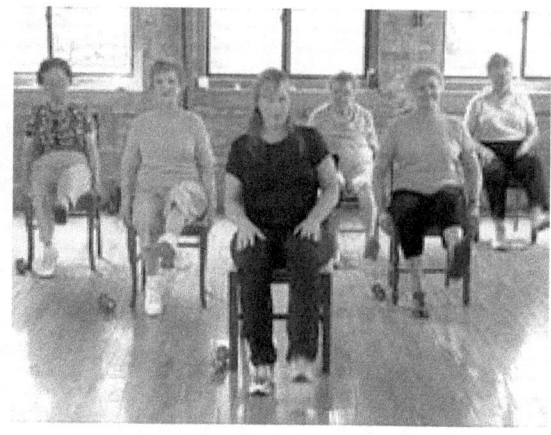

Examples of chair cardio exercises include seated jumping jacks, chair marches, and seated high knees. These exercises can help to improve cardiovascular health, endurance, and overall fitness, while also building strength and flexibility in the lower body.

One of the advantages of chair cardio is that it can be performed in a small space, making it a convenient option for home workouts. It can also be modified to suit different fitness levels, allowing individuals to gradually increase the intensity of their workouts over time.

When performing chair cardio exercises, it is important to use proper form and technique to avoid injury. It is also important to start slowly and gradually increase the intensity of the workout as fitness levels improve.

Chair cardio exercises are a great way to increase heart rate and get the blood flowing without putting too much stress on the body. It is an ideal option for individuals who want to start exercising but have limited mobility or are not ready for high-impact activities.

Chair cardio exercises can be done by anyone, regardless of fitness level or age. It is also a great way to add variety to your exercise routine, as there are many different exercises that can be performed while sitting in a chair.

Some of the benefits of chair cardio exercises include improved cardiovascular health, better circulation, increased energy levels, and improved muscle tone. These exercises can also be effective in reducing stress and improving overall mood.

To get the most out of chair cardio exercises, it is important to perform them consistently and to gradually increase the intensity of the workout. It is also important to pay attention to proper form and technique to avoid injury.

Some examples of chair cardio exercises include seated arm circles, seated high kicks, seated leg extensions, and seated twists. These exercises can be modified to suit different fitness levels and can be performed with or without additional equipment such as dumbbells or resistance bands.

Overall, chair cardio exercises are a great way to improve fitness and well-being for individuals with frailty syndrome or limited mobility. They provide a low-impact workout that can be easily modified to suit individual needs and fitness levels.

Chapter 4

Flexibility and Mobility

Flexibility and mobility are important components of a well-rounded exercise routine, especially for individuals with frailty syndrome. These exercises can help improve range of motion, reduce the risk of injury, and improve overall physical function.

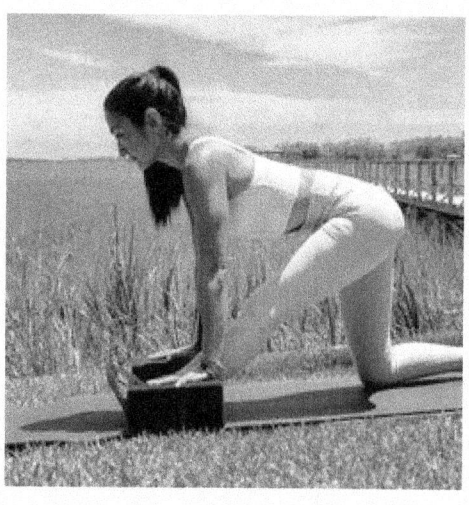

Flexibility exercises involve stretching the muscles and joints to improve range of motion and reduce stiffness. These exercises can be performed before and after a workout to help prepare the body and reduce the risk of injury.

Mobility exercises involve movements that simulate daily activities such as walking, reaching, and bending. These exercises can help improve balance, coordination, and overall physical function.

Examples of flexibility exercises include static stretches such as hamstring stretches, quad stretches, and calf stretches. Dynamic stretching exercises can also be incorporated into a routine, such as leg swings, walking lunges, and arm circles.

Mobility exercises can include movements such as squats, lunges, and step-ups, as well as exercises that focus on balance such as single-leg balance and heel-toe walking.

It is important to perform flexibility and mobility exercises regularly, but it is also important to listen to your body and avoid overstretching or pushing too hard. Gradually increasing the intensity and duration of these exercises can help improve flexibility and mobility over time.

In addition to improving physical function and reducing the risk of injury, flexibility and mobility exercises can also have mental health benefits. These exercises can help reduce stress and tension in the body, promote relaxation, and improve overall mood and wellbeing.

For individuals with frailty syndrome, it is important to work with a healthcare provider or qualified exercise professional to develop an exercise routine that is safe and effective. It is also important to properly warm up before engaging in flexibility and mobility exercises to prevent injury.

Incorporating these exercises into a regular routine can be done in a variety of ways, such as incorporating them into a warm-up or cool-down routine or dedicating a specific time during the day for stretching and mobility exercises.

Overall, incorporating flexibility and mobility exercises into a regular exercise routine can help improve physical function, reduce the risk of injury, and improve overall wellbeing for individuals with frailty syndrome.

Yoga

Yoga is a form of exercise that combines physical postures, breathing techniques, and meditation to promote overall health and wellbeing. It has been shown to have numerous benefits for individuals with frailty syndrome, including improved flexibility, balance, strength, and mental health.

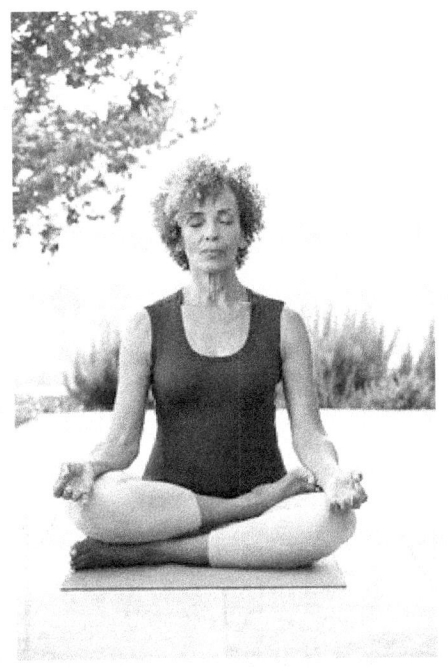

Yoga can be adapted to accommodate individuals with different levels of ability and mobility, making it an excellent option for those with frailty syndrome. Modifications can be made to the postures and movements to accommodate individuals with mobility or balance challenges, and props such as blocks, straps, or chairs can be used to provide support.

Practicing yoga regularly can also help reduce stress and anxiety, improve sleep quality, and promote a sense of relaxation and calmness. It can be practiced in a group setting or individually, and there are many resources available online and in-person to learn and practice yoga.

However, it is important for individuals with frailty syndrome to work with a qualified yoga instructor or healthcare provider to ensure that the practice is safe and appropriate for their needs. Certain postures or movements may need to be modified or avoided altogether, and it is important to listen to the body and avoid pushing beyond one's limits.

There are many different types of yoga, each with its own focus and style. Some styles of yoga, such as Hatha or Restorative yoga, may be particularly beneficial for individuals with frailty syndrome as they focus on gentle movements, relaxation, and breathwork.

Chair yoga is another option that can be particularly beneficial for individuals with mobility or balance challenges. Chair yoga incorporates many of the same principles as traditional yoga, but uses a chair for support and stability. This can make the practice more accessible and help individuals build strength and flexibility at their own pace.

In addition to physical benefits, yoga can also provide emotional and mental benefits for individuals with frailty syndrome. Research has shown that practicing yoga regularly can help reduce symptoms of depression and anxiety, improve mood, and increase feelings of wellbeing.

It is important to note that while yoga can be a safe and effective exercise option for individuals with frailty syndrome, it should not be used as a replacement for medical treatment or advice from a healthcare provider. Individuals should always consult with their doctor or a qualified yoga instructor before starting a new exercise program.

Pilates

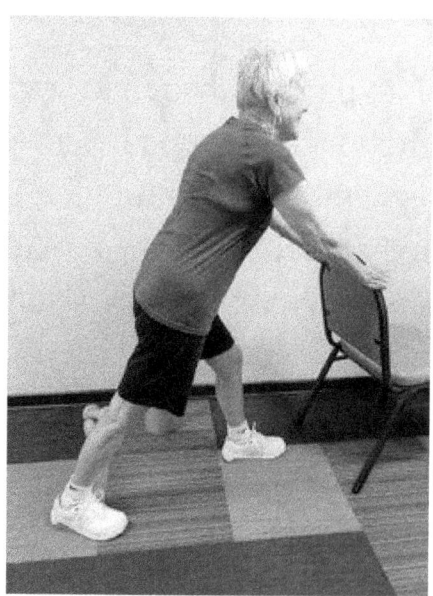

Pilates is a low-impact exercise that can help individuals with frailty syndrome build strength, flexibility, and balance. Pilates exercises are typically done on a mat or with specialized equipment, such as a Pilates reformer or Cadillac machine.

One of the key principles of Pilates is engaging the core muscles, which can help improve posture, balance, and stability. Pilates exercises also incorporate a focus on breathing and mind-body connection, which can help reduce stress and promote relaxation.

Pilates exercises can be modified to accommodate individuals with different levels of ability and mobility, making it a versatile exercise option for individuals with frailty syndrome. Some Pilates exercises, such as the Pilates hundred or pelvic tilt, can be done lying down, while others, such as the

Pilates side kick or plank, can be done in a seated or standing position.

Pilates is a gentle yet effective form of exercise that can be particularly beneficial for individuals with frailty syndrome. It is a form of exercise that can be done in a group setting or one-on-one with a trained instructor, making it a social activity that can help improve mental health and wellbeing as well.

Regular Pilates practice can improve overall flexibility and range of motion, which can reduce the risk of falls and other injuries. It can also help to alleviate back pain and joint stiffness, common symptoms of frailty syndrome. Additionally, Pilates can help to build strength in the legs, hips, and core, which are important muscle groups for maintaining balance and stability.

Pilates is a low-impact exercise, meaning that it places minimal stress on the joints and can be a safe option for individuals with frailty syndrome who may be more prone to injuries or pain. Many Pilates exercises can also be modified to be done in a seated position, making it accessible for individuals with limited mobility.

As with any exercise program, it is important to consult with a healthcare provider or a qualified Pilates instructor before starting a new routine, especially if you have any health concerns or injuries.

Tai Chi

Tai Chi is a form of Chinese martial arts that is often practiced for its health benefits. It involves a series of slow and graceful movements that are coordinated with deep breathing and mental focus. Tai Chi has been shown to have numerous benefits for individuals with frailty syndrome.

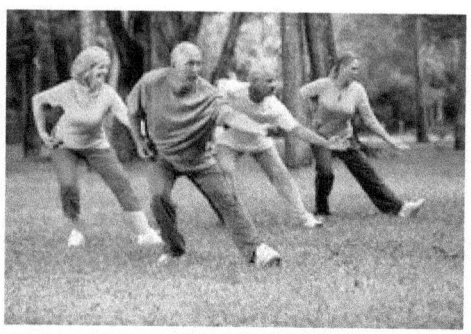

One of the main benefits of Tai Chi is improved balance and coordination. The slow, controlled movements of Tai Chi can help to strengthen the muscles used for balance and stability, reducing the risk of falls and injuries. Tai Chi has also been shown to improve flexibility and range of motion, which can help to reduce joint stiffness and pain.

In addition to its physical benefits, Tai Chi can also have a positive impact on mental health and wellbeing. It has been shown to reduce stress and anxiety, improve mood, and promote better sleep. For individuals with frailty syndrome who may be dealing with other health issues, Tai Chi can be a helpful tool for managing symptoms and improving overall quality of life.

While Tai Chi is generally considered a safe form of exercise, it's important for individuals with frailty syndrome to consult with their healthcare provider before starting a Tai Chi program. Depending on an individual's specific health needs and abilities, modifications may be necessary to ensure safety and prevent injury.

For individuals with limited mobility or balance issues, seated Tai Chi may be a more appropriate option. This involves performing Tai Chi movements while sitting in a chair, which can help to reduce the risk of falls and make the exercise more accessible.

Tai Chi classes are widely available at community centers, senior centers, and fitness studios, and can be a great way to get started with this beneficial form of exercise. Some classes may be specifically designed for individuals with frailty syndrome or other health conditions, and may offer modifications and additional support.

In addition to in-person classes, there are also many online resources and instructional videos available for practicing Tai Chi at home. As with any form of exercise, it's important to start slowly and gradually build up intensity and duration over time. With consistency and patience, Tai Chi can be a valuable tool for improving strength, balance, and overall wellbeing in individuals with frailty syndrome.

Stretching

Stretching is an important component of any exercise program, as it helps to improve flexibility and range of motion, prevent injury, and promote relaxation. For individuals with frailty syndrome, incorporating regular stretching into their exercise routine can be especially beneficial for maintaining mobility and reducing the risk of falls.

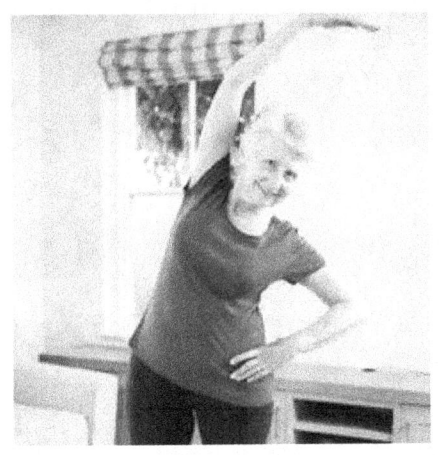

Before beginning any stretching routine, it's important to warm up the muscles with a few minutes of light activity, such as walking or gentle movements. This can help to increase blood flow and prepare the muscles for stretching.

There are many different types of stretches that can be beneficial for individuals with frailty syndrome, including:

1. Static stretching: This involves holding a stretch in a fixed position for a period of time, typically around 30 seconds. Static stretching can be useful for improving flexibility and range of motion in specific muscle groups.
2. Dynamic stretching: This involves moving the body through a range of motion repeatedly, such as with arm circles or leg swings. Dynamic stretching can help to improve mobility

and prepare the body for more intense activity.

3. Proprioceptive neuromuscular facilitation (PNF) stretching: This involves contracting and relaxing the muscles while stretching, typically with the assistance of a partner or resistance band. PNF stretching can help to improve flexibility and range of motion in a shorter amount of time than static stretching alone.

It's important to listen to your body and not push past your limits when stretching. Stretching should not cause pain or discomfort, and if you experience any pain or discomfort, it's important to stop and consult with a healthcare provider.

The Frailty Fighter

Chapter 5

Creating a Personalized Exercise Plan

Creating a personalized exercise plan is essential to combatting frailty syndrome. It allows you to tailor your workouts to your specific needs and abilities, ensuring that you are getting the most out of your exercise routine. When creating your plan, it's important to take into account your current level of fitness, any health concerns or limitations, and your goals.

Start by setting specific, measurable goals that you want to achieve through exercise. These goals could include increasing strength, improving balance, or increasing cardiovascular endurance. Once you have identified your goals, you can begin to create a plan that will help you achieve them.

When creating your plan, be sure to include a variety of exercises that target different areas of the body and different types of exercise (e.g., strength training, cardiovascular exercise, flexibility/mobility). It's also important to gradually increase the intensity and duration of your workouts over time to avoid injury and continue to challenge yourself.

Consulting with a healthcare professional or certified fitness trainer can be helpful in creating a personalized exercise plan. They can provide guidance on proper technique, modifications for any limitations or health concerns, and help track progress towards your goals.

Additionally, it's important to consider your schedule and availability when creating your exercise plan. Choose a time of day that works best for you and your lifestyle, and aim to exercise at least three to four times per week. It's also important to listen to your body and make adjustments as necessary. If you experience pain or discomfort during exercise, it's important to rest and modify your routine to avoid further injury.

Incorporating social support can also be helpful in sticking to your exercise plan. Consider joining a fitness class or finding a workout partner to help keep you motivated and accountable.

Finally, don't forget to track your progress and celebrate your successes along the way. Keeping a workout journal or using a fitness tracking app can help you stay on track and see the progress you are making towards your goals.

Creating a personalized exercise plan takes time and effort, but the benefits are well worth it. By committing to regular exercise and tailoring your routine to your specific needs, you can improve your strength, balance, and overall health, and combat the effects of frailty syndrome.

Assessing Your Fitness Level

Before beginning any exercise program, it's important to assess your current fitness level. This will help you determine where you are starting from, and set realistic goals for your exercise plan.

There are several different methods you can use to assess your fitness level, including:

1. Cardiovascular fitness test: This measures how well your heart and lungs function during exercise. You can use a step test or a timed walk test to assess your cardiovascular fitness.
2. Strength test: This measures your muscular strength and endurance. You can use bodyweight exercises or weightlifting to assess your strength.
3. Flexibility test: This measures your range of motion in your joints. You can use simple stretches or yoga poses to assess your flexibility.
4. Balance test: This measures your ability to maintain your balance during different movements. You can use exercises such as standing on one leg or

walking heel-to-toe to assess your balance.

Once you have assessed your fitness level, you can use this information to set realistic goals for your exercise plan. For example, if you have low cardiovascular fitness, you may want to focus on cardio exercises such as walking or cycling. If you have weak muscles, you may want to focus on strength training exercises.

Remember, fitness is a journey, not a destination. Your fitness level will change over time as you continue to exercise and improve your health. By assessing your fitness level and setting realistic goals, you can create an exercise plan that will help you reach your full potential and combat the effects of frailty syndrome.

Developing a Plan that Fits Your Needs

Creating a personalized exercise plan requires an understanding of your current fitness level and your health status. Before you start any new exercise routine, it is important to assess your fitness level and consult with your healthcare provider.

Assessing your fitness level may involve a series of tests and measurements such as a body composition analysis, cardiovascular endurance test, muscular strength and endurance test, and flexibility assessment. These tests can help you determine your current fitness level and identify areas where you need improvement.

After assessing your fitness level, it is important to develop a plan that fits your needs and goals. Your plan should include exercises that address your areas of weakness and help you achieve your fitness goals. It should also take into account your preferences, available time, and any health conditions or physical limitations.

When developing your plan, consider the following:

- Frequency: How often will you exercise? Aim for at least 3-5 days per week.
- Intensity: How hard will you exercise? Choose exercises that challenge you but don't cause pain or discomfort.
- Time: How long will you exercise? Aim for at least 30 minutes per session.
- Type: What types of exercises will you do? Choose a variety of exercises that work different muscle groups and address different aspects of fitness, such as strength, endurance, and flexibility.

- Progression: How will you progress over time? Gradually increase the intensity, duration, and frequency of your workouts as your fitness level improves.

Remember to listen to your body and adjust your plan as needed. With a personalized exercise plan, you can combat frailty syndrome and improve your overall health and well-being.

Tracking Progress and Making Adjustments

Tracking your progress is crucial to ensure that your exercise plan is effective and to identify areas where adjustments may be needed. You can use various tools to track your progress, including fitness apps, wearable fitness trackers, or a simple pen and paper.

Start by setting realistic goals and tracking your progress towards achieving them. This can include tracking your weight, body measurements, and fitness milestones such as the amount of weight you can lift or the distance you can run.

As you progress, you may need to adjust your exercise plan to continue challenging yourself and seeing results. This could involve increasing the duration or intensity of your workouts or incorporating new exercises to target different muscle groups.

It's also important to listen to your body and make adjustments as needed to prevent injury and avoid overtraining. If you experience pain or discomfort during exercise, consult with your healthcare provider or a certified fitness professional for guidance on how to modify your exercise plan.

Remember, developing a personalized exercise plan takes time and patience, but the benefits of combating frailty syndrome are worth the effort. With consistency and dedication, you can build strength, improve balance and coordination, and enhance your overall physical health and well-being.

Tracking your progress and making adjustments to your exercise plan is essential for combating frailty syndrome. Regularly monitoring your progress will allow you to see improvements and identify areas where you need to focus your efforts. It will also help you stay motivated and on track with your goals.

There are many different ways to track your progress, including keeping a workout journal, using a fitness app or tracker, or working with a personal trainer. Whichever method you choose, it's important to track both quantitative data (such as weight, body fat percentage, and number of repetitions) and qualitative data (such as how you feel during and after exercise).

As you progress, you may need to adjust your exercise plan to continue making gains. This could mean increasing the weight or resistance of your exercises, changing up your routine to challenge your body in new ways, or adding new exercises to target specific areas.

It's important to listen to your body and make adjustments as needed. If you experience pain or discomfort during exercise, it may be a sign that you need to dial back the intensity or modify your movements. It's also important to consult with your doctor or a qualified fitness professional before making any significant changes to your exercise plan.

Chapter 6

Staying Motivated and Focused

Staying motivated and focused can be challenging when it comes to exercise, especially for individuals with frailty syndrome. However, there are several strategies that can be used to stay on track and reach your goals:

1. Set realistic goals: Make sure your goals are attainable and measurable. Set small, achievable goals and celebrate your successes along the way.
2. Find a workout buddy: Having a partner to exercise with can make the experience more enjoyable and hold you accountable.

3. Mix it up: Try different types of exercise to keep things interesting and prevent boredom.

4. Reward yourself: Treat yourself when you reach milestones or achieve your goals. This can help you stay motivated and focused.

5. Track your progress: Keep a journal or use a fitness tracking app to monitor your progress. Seeing improvements in your fitness level can be a great motivator.

6. Stay positive: Remember that setbacks are normal and part of the process. Don't be too hard on yourself and focus on the progress you've made.

By using these strategies, you can stay motivated and focused on your exercise plan, leading to improved health and a higher quality of life.

Overcoming Challenges

Overcoming challenges is an essential part of any exercise routine, especially for individuals with frailty syndrome. Some of the common challenges that may arise include fatigue, joint pain, muscle soreness, and lack of motivation.

To overcome fatigue, it is essential to ensure that you get enough rest and sleep. It is also essential to fuel your body with healthy foods and stay hydrated throughout the day. Incorporating strength training exercises into your routine can also help reduce fatigue and build endurance over time.

Joint pain and muscle soreness can be addressed through proper warm-up and stretching techniques. It is also important to listen to your body and adjust your exercise routine as needed to avoid overexertion. Low-impact exercises like swimming, cycling, and chair cardio can also be helpful for reducing joint pain and muscle soreness.

Lack of motivation can be a significant barrier to sticking to an exercise routine. It is important to identify your personal motivations for exercising and remind yourself of them regularly. Setting achievable goals and tracking progress can also help you stay motivated and focused.

In some cases, working with a certified personal trainer or physical therapist may be necessary to address specific challenges and develop an exercise plan that is safe and effective for your individual needs.

Finding Support

While exercise can be a great way to boost your physical and mental health, it can also be a challenge to stick with a routine on your own. Finding support from others can be an effective way to stay motivated and on track with your exercise goals.

Here are some ways to find support:

1. Join a group fitness class: Group fitness classes are a great way to meet like-minded individuals who are also interested in exercise. These classes can be found at local gyms, community centers, or online.
2. Work with a personal trainer: A personal trainer can provide one-on-one support and motivation. They can also help you develop a personalized exercise plan based on your specific needs and goals.

3. Join an exercise group or club: There are many local exercise groups and clubs that you can join, such as running or cycling clubs. These groups provide social support and can be a great way to make new friends while staying active.

4. Use social media: Social media platforms like Facebook and Instagram can provide access to fitness communities and support groups. Following fitness influencers or joining online groups can help keep you motivated and connected with others who share your interests.

5. Find a workout buddy: Partnering up with a friend or family member who shares your interest in exercise can be a great way to stay accountable and motivated. Scheduling regular workouts together can help you both stay on track with your exercise goals.

Remember, finding support is an important part of staying committed to your exercise routine. Don't be afraid to reach out and connect with others who share your interest in physical activity.

Incorporating Exercise into Your Daily Routine

Many people struggle to find time to exercise, but it is important to make it a priority for your health and well-being. Here are some tips to help you make exercise a part of your daily routine:

1. Schedule it: Just like you would schedule a meeting or appointment, schedule time for exercise in your daily calendar. This will make it a priority and remind you to do it.
2. Choose an activity you enjoy: If you choose an activity you enjoy, you are

more likely to stick with it. This could be anything from walking to yoga to dancing. Find something that brings you joy and makes you feel good.

3. Make it social: Exercise with a friend or family member to make it more enjoyable and hold each other accountable.

4. Take breaks at work: If you have a sedentary job, take breaks throughout the day to get up and move. This could be as simple as taking a walk around the office or doing some stretches.

5. Multitask: Find ways to incorporate exercise into your daily activities. For example, you could do squats while brushing your teeth or take the stairs instead of the elevator.

6. Be flexible: Don't beat yourself up if you miss a day of exercise. Life happens, and it's important to be

flexible and adjust your routine as needed.

By incorporating exercise into your daily routine, you can improve your overall health and well-being. Remember to start small and gradually increase your activity level over time.

Making Healthy Lifestyle Choices

Making healthy lifestyle choices is an essential part of managing frailty syndrome. Exercise alone cannot combat this condition without a comprehensive approach to healthy living. Making healthy choices includes adopting a balanced and nutritious diet, avoiding harmful substances such as tobacco and excessive alcohol consumption, getting adequate rest and sleep, managing stress, and maintaining social connections.

Eating a balanced diet that is rich in fruits, vegetables, whole grains, lean proteins, and healthy fats can provide the body with essential nutrients needed for optimal health. Avoiding unhealthy substances such as tobacco and excessive alcohol consumption can help prevent or manage various health conditions that can exacerbate frailty syndrome. Getting adequate rest and sleep can help reduce fatigue and improve overall physical and mental health. Managing stress through relaxation techniques, mindfulness practices, or therapy can improve mental health and reduce the risk of various chronic diseases.

Maintaining social connections is also crucial to combat frailty syndrome, as social isolation and loneliness can contribute to the worsening of this condition. Engaging in social activities, participating in community events, or joining a support group can help combat feelings of loneliness and social isolation.

Making healthy lifestyle choices is crucial in preventing and managing frailty syndrome. In addition to exercise, there are several other factors that can contribute to overall health and well-being, including nutrition, sleep, stress management, and social connection.

A balanced diet rich in nutrients can help provide the energy and nourishment needed to maintain physical function and support a healthy immune system. It is important to consume a variety of foods from all food groups, including fruits, vegetables, whole grains, lean protein, and healthy fats.

Getting adequate sleep is also important in promoting physical and mental health. Lack of sleep can lead to fatigue, decreased immune function, and impaired cognitive abilities, making it more difficult to engage in exercise and other activities.

Managing stress is another important aspect of a healthy lifestyle. Chronic stress can have negative effects on physical and mental health, contributing to conditions such as hypertension, heart disease, and depression. Engaging in stress-reducing activities such as meditation, yoga, or mindfulness practices can help promote relaxation and reduce stress levels.

Finally, social connection and engagement can also have a positive impact on overall health and well-being. Loneliness and social isolation have been linked to an increased risk of chronic health conditions and a decline in physical function. Staying connected with friends and family, joining a community group or club, or volunteering can all help promote social connection and support overall health.

By making healthy lifestyle choices and incorporating exercise into a daily routine, individuals can help prevent and manage frailty syndrome and promote overall health and well-being.

The Frailty Fighter

Chapter 7

Exercise Modifications for Special Considerations

Exercise modifications for special consideration refer to adapting exercise routines to meet the specific needs of individuals with health conditions that require unique considerations. Some health conditions that may require exercise modifications include:

1. Arthritis: People with arthritis may require modifications to their exercise routine to avoid putting stress on the joints. Low-impact exercises such as swimming or cycling may be recommended.

2. Diabetes: Exercise can help manage blood sugar levels in people with diabetes, but they may need to adjust their medication and monitor their blood sugar more closely during physical activity.

3. Heart disease: People with heart disease may need to start with low-intensity exercises and gradually increase the intensity and duration over time. They may also need to monitor their heart rate and blood pressure during exercise.

4. Osteoporosis: People with osteoporosis may need to avoid exercises that put too much stress on the bones, such as high-impact exercises. Resistance training and weight-bearing exercises may be recommended.

5. Chronic obstructive pulmonary disease (COPD): People with COPD may need to start with exercises that are less intense and gradually increase the intensity over time. They may also need to use supplemental oxygen during exercise.

6. Pregnancy: Pregnant women may need to modify their exercise routine to avoid certain exercises that may harm the baby. Low-impact exercises such as walking or prenatal yoga may be recommended.

By making modifications to exercise routines, individuals with special health considerations can still benefit from physical activity while reducing the risk of injury or exacerbating their health condition. It is important to consult with a healthcare provider or qualified exercise professional before beginning an exercise routine, especially if you have a health condition that requires special consideration.

Exercises for those with Arthritis

Arthritis is a common condition that affects many individuals, especially as they age. This condition can cause joint pain, stiffness, and limited mobility, making exercise difficult. However, exercise is crucial for individuals with arthritis to maintain strength and flexibility, reduce pain and inflammation, and improve overall quality of life.

Here are some exercises that can be modified to suit the needs of individuals with arthritis:

1. Low-impact aerobic exercise: Walking, cycling, and swimming are all great

forms of low-impact aerobic exercise that can be modified for individuals with arthritis. These exercises are easy on the joints and can help improve cardiovascular health.

2. Strength training: Strength training can help improve muscle strength, which can help protect the joints and reduce pain. Resistance bands and light weights can be used for strength training exercises, and modifications can be made to accommodate any joint pain or limited mobility.

3. Yoga and Pilates: These exercises can help improve flexibility, balance, and strength, all of which can help reduce joint pain and stiffness. Modifications can be made to accommodate any joint pain or limited mobility.

4. Water exercises: Water exercise is a low-impact exercise that can be particularly helpful for individuals with

arthritis. The buoyancy of the water can help reduce joint pain and stiffness, making it easier to exercise.

5. Tai Chi: Tai Chi is a gentle exercise that can help improve balance and flexibility, reduce stress, and improve overall well-being. Modifications can be made to accommodate any joint pain or limited mobility.

It's important to consult with a healthcare professional before starting any new exercise program, particularly if you have arthritis. They can help you determine which exercises are safe and effective for your specific needs and limitations.

Exercises for those with Osteoporosis

When designing an exercise program for individuals with osteoporosis, it is essential to consider the potential risk of falls and fractures due to weakened bones. Therefore, low-impact exercises that do not put excessive stress on the bones are recommended. Here are some exercises that can be helpful for individuals with osteoporosis:

1. Walking: Walking is a weight-bearing exercise that helps to strengthen bones and improve overall health. It is a low-impact exercise that is safe and easy to do.
2. Tai chi: Tai chi is a gentle form of exercise that involves slow and controlled movements. It can help to improve balance and coordination, which can reduce the risk of falls.
3. Yoga: Yoga is a low-impact exercise that can help to improve flexibility, balance, and strength. It can be modified to suit different levels of fitness and abilities.

4. Resistance training: Resistance training with light weights or resistance bands can help to improve bone density and muscle strength. However, it is important to avoid exercises that involve twisting or bending the spine.

5. Swimming: Swimming is a non-weight-bearing exercise that is easy on the joints and can help to improve overall fitness and flexibility.

Before starting any exercise program, individuals with osteoporosis should consult with their healthcare provider to ensure that the exercises are safe and appropriate for their condition.

Exercises for those with Joint Replacements

joint replacements, such as hip or knee replacements, can limit mobility and range of motion, but exercise can help to maintain and improve joint function. It's important to talk to your doctor and physical therapist before beginning any exercise program after a joint replacement surgery. Here are some exercises that may be helpful:

1. Range-of-motion exercises: These exercises involve moving the joint through its full range of motion. Examples include ankle pumps, knee bends, and hip rotations.
2. Strengthening exercises: These exercises can help to improve muscle strength and support the joint. Examples include leg presses, calf raises, and hip abductions.

3. Low-impact aerobics: Exercises such as walking, cycling, and swimming can help to improve cardiovascular health and overall fitness without putting too much stress on the joints.

4. Resistance band exercises: Resistance bands can be used to strengthen the muscles around the joint without putting too much stress on the joint itself. Examples include leg extensions, hip adductions, and knee curls.

It's important to start with low-impact exercises and gradually increase the intensity and duration of your workouts as your joint heals and strengthens. Always listen to your body and stop if you feel pain or discomfort.

Exercises for those with Chronic Pain

Chronic pain can make exercise challenging, but it is still important for maintaining physical and mental health. However, it is essential to approach exercise with caution and work with a healthcare professional to develop a safe and effective exercise plan.

Some low-impact exercises that may be beneficial for those with chronic pain include:

1. Yoga: Yoga combines physical postures, breathing techniques, and meditation to help reduce stress and relieve pain.
2. Tai Chi: Tai Chi is a gentle form of exercise that involves slow, flowing movements and deep breathing. It can help improve flexibility, balance, and reduce stress.
3. Aquatic exercise: Water provides buoyancy and support, making it an ideal environment for exercise. Swimming, water aerobics, and other aquatic exercises can help improve

cardiovascular fitness, strength, and flexibility while minimizing joint impact.

4. Walking: Walking is a low-impact exercise that can help improve cardiovascular fitness and strengthen muscles. It is also an excellent way to reduce stress and boost mood.

5. Cycling: Cycling is a low-impact exercise that can help improve cardiovascular fitness and strength. Stationary bikes are a great option for those who experience pain with outdoor cycling.

It is important to start slowly and gradually increase the intensity and duration of exercise over time. It is also crucial to listen to your body and stop any exercise that causes pain or discomfort. Working with a healthcare professional and a certified exercise professional can help ensure that you are exercising safely and effectively.

The Frailty Fighter

Chapter 8

Nutrition and Hydration

Nutrition and hydration are important components of a healthy lifestyle and can greatly impact one's ability to exercise and combat frailty syndrome. Eating a well-balanced diet rich in nutrients can provide the necessary energy and nutrients for the body to function optimally. Adequate hydration is also important to ensure proper body functioning and prevent dehydration, which can lead to fatigue, dizziness, and other health complications.

When preparing a meal plan, it is important to consider the individual's specific needs and dietary restrictions. For example, individuals with certain medical conditions such as diabetes or heart disease may need to follow a specific diet plan. Additionally, older adults may have different nutritional requirements than younger individuals due to changes in metabolism and body composition.

In general, a healthy diet should include a variety of fruits, vegetables, whole grains, lean protein sources, and healthy fats. Limiting processed foods, sugary drinks, and high-fat foods can also improve overall health.

Hydration is also crucial, especially during exercise. It is recommended that individuals drink water before, during, and after exercise to prevent dehydration. Older adults may have a decreased sense of thirst, so it is important to drink water regularly throughout the day, even if not feeling thirsty.

Nutrition and hydration play a crucial role in exercise performance and overall health. The food and drinks we consume provide the necessary fuel for our bodies to function optimally during physical activity, and help to support muscle growth and repair, improve endurance, and reduce the risk of injury.

Proper nutrition is important both before and after exercise. Before exercising, it's important to fuel up with a balanced meal that includes carbohydrates, protein, and healthy fats. Carbohydrates provide energy for physical activity, while protein helps to build and repair muscle tissue. Healthy fats help to provide sustained energy throughout the workout. Good pre-workout meal options include oatmeal with berries and nuts, a turkey and avocado sandwich on whole grain bread, or a fruit and yogurt smoothie.

After exercising, it's important to replenish the body with a combination of carbohydrates and protein. This helps to restore energy levels and support muscle recovery. Good post-workout meal options include a grilled chicken breast with sweet potato and vegetables, a quinoa and vegetable stir-fry with tofu, or a salmon and avocado salad.

Staying hydrated is also crucial for exercise performance and overall health. Water helps to regulate body temperature, transport nutrients and oxygen to the muscles, and remove waste products from the body. It's important to drink plenty of water before, during, and after exercise, and to replenish electrolytes lost through sweating with sports drinks or electrolyte supplements if necessary.

Overall, a balanced and nutritious diet that includes plenty of fruits, vegetables, whole grains, lean protein, and healthy fats is essential for optimal exercise performance and overall health.

Healthy Eating Habits for Aging Adults

As people age, their nutritional needs and dietary requirements may change. It is important for aging adults to maintain a healthy diet to support overall health, prevent chronic disease, and support their exercise routine. Here are some healthy eating habits that aging adults can adopt:

1. Focus on nutrient-dense foods: Choose foods that are rich in nutrients, such as fruits, vegetables, whole grains, lean proteins, and healthy fats.
2. Stay hydrated: Drink plenty of water and other hydrating fluids to maintain proper hydration. As people age, their sense of thirst may decrease, so it is important to drink water regularly throughout the day.
3. Eat smaller, more frequent meals: Eating smaller, more frequent meals can help maintain steady energy levels and prevent overeating.
4. Limit processed and high-sugar foods: Processed and high-sugar foods can lead to inflammation, weight gain, and other health problems. Limiting these

foods and choosing whole, unprocessed options is a healthier choice.

5. Consider supplements: Aging adults may have trouble getting all of their necessary nutrients through their diet alone. Consider talking to a healthcare professional about adding supplements to your daily routine.

6. Avoid skipping meals: Skipping meals can lead to overeating and unhealthy food choices later in the day. Eating regularly throughout the day can help maintain energy levels and support overall health.

7. Pay attention to food safety: As people age, their immune systems may weaken, making them more susceptible to foodborne illnesses. Pay attention to food safety practices, such as properly storing and cooking foods, to prevent illness.

Hydration Guidelines for Aging Adults

As we age, our body's ability to conserve water decreases. This means that older adults may not feel as thirsty as they once did, which can lead to dehydration. Dehydration can cause a host of problems, including fatigue, dizziness, confusion, and kidney problems. It's essential for aging adults to stay hydrated, especially when exercising.

The National Academies of Sciences, Engineering, and Medicine recommends that men drink about 3.7 liters (125 ounces) of fluids per day, and women drink about 2.7 liters (91 ounces) of fluids per day. This includes fluids from all sources, such as water, milk, juice, coffee, and tea. However, these recommendations are for sedentary adults and may need to be adjusted based on activity level and climate.

When exercising, it's crucial to drink enough fluids to replace the water lost through sweating. A general rule of thumb is to drink 17-20 ounces of water 2-3 hours before exercising, 8 ounces of water 20-30 minutes before exercising, and 7-10 ounces of water every 10-20 minutes during exercise.

It's also important to remember that thirst is not always a reliable indicator of hydration status, especially for aging adults. Therefore, it's a good idea to drink water regularly throughout the day, even if you don't feel thirsty. Additionally, foods with high water content, such as fruits and vegetables, can also contribute to overall hydration.

The Frailty Fighter

Chapter 9

Mental Health and Exercise

Exercise is not only beneficial for physical health, but it can also have a positive impact on mental health. Regular exercise has been shown to reduce symptoms of depression, anxiety, and stress, as well as improve mood and overall well-being.

One theory suggests that exercise helps to release endorphins, which are natural chemicals in the body that promote feelings of happiness and pleasure. Exercise can also provide a sense of accomplishment and boost self-confidence, which can help to combat negative thoughts and emotions.

In addition, exercise can provide a distraction from daily stressors and give individuals a sense of control over their lives. Engaging in physical activity with others can also provide social support and a sense of community, which can be particularly important for those experiencing loneliness or isolation.

The Connection Between Exercise and Mental Health

There is a strong connection between exercise and mental health. Physical activity has been shown to have numerous benefits for mental health, including reducing symptoms of anxiety and depression, improving mood and self-esteem, and reducing stress. Exercise can also improve cognitive function and overall brain health, including memory and attention.

One of the main ways exercise can improve mental health is by releasing endorphins, which are natural chemicals in the brain that act as painkillers and mood elevators. Endorphins can help reduce feelings of anxiety and depression and improve overall mood.

Exercise can also provide a sense of accomplishment and boost self-esteem, especially when progress is made in fitness levels or achieving fitness goals. Additionally, exercise can serve as a healthy coping mechanism for stress, providing a physical outlet for pent-up emotions and tension.

Regular exercise can also improve sleep, which is essential for good mental health. Poor sleep has been linked to increased risk of anxiety and depression.

Research has shown that regular exercise can have a positive impact on mental health, including reducing symptoms of anxiety and depression, improving mood and self-esteem, and promoting overall well-being. Exercise can also provide a sense of accomplishment and boost self-confidence, leading to a more positive outlook on life.

The reasons for these benefits are complex and not yet fully understood, but it is believed that exercise helps to regulate levels of neurotransmitters such as serotonin and dopamine, which are important for mood regulation. Exercise can also reduce levels of stress hormones like cortisol and promote the release of endorphins, which are natural mood enhancers.

In addition to the chemical effects, exercise can also provide a sense of social support and community through group fitness classes or sports teams. This can lead to feelings of connectedness and reduce feelings of loneliness and isolation.

It is important to note that exercise should not be considered a replacement for professional mental health treatment, but rather as a complementary therapy. It is always recommended to consult with a healthcare professional before starting a new exercise routine or making significant changes to an existing one.

Reducing Stress and Anxiety Through Exercise

Exercise is an effective way to reduce stress and anxiety. It is a natural stress reliever that helps reduce tension, increase relaxation, and improve mood. When you exercise, your body releases endorphins, which are hormones that create feelings of happiness and euphoria. These endorphins can help reduce stress and anxiety and improve your overall mental well-being.

Aerobic exercise, in particular, has been found to be effective in reducing stress and anxiety. This includes activities such as jogging, cycling, swimming, or dancing. Aerobic exercise increases blood flow to the brain and helps reduce the levels of stress hormones in the body.

In addition to aerobic exercise, mind-body exercises such as yoga and tai chi can also help reduce stress and anxiety. These practices combine physical movement with mindfulness and meditation techniques, which can help calm the mind and reduce stress.

Resistance training, or weightlifting, can also be an effective way to reduce stress and anxiety. This type of exercise helps increase feelings of strength and confidence, which can improve self-esteem and reduce feelings of stress.

Stress and anxiety are common problems that many people face, and exercise can be an effective way to reduce these negative feelings. When we exercise, our body releases endorphins, which are natural chemicals that help to reduce stress and improve mood.

In addition to the release of endorphins, exercise can also help to reduce levels of the stress hormone cortisol. High levels of cortisol in the body can lead to a range of negative health effects, including weight gain, high blood pressure, and a weakened immune system. By reducing cortisol levels through exercise, we can help to protect our bodies from these negative effects.

Another way that exercise can help to reduce stress and anxiety is by providing a sense of control and accomplishment. When we set and achieve exercise goals, we feel a sense of satisfaction and accomplishment that can help to improve our mood and reduce stress.

Exercise can also provide a healthy distraction from the stressors of daily life. By focusing on our physical activity, we can take our minds off of the things that are causing us stress and anxiety.

Finally, exercise can provide an opportunity for social interaction and support, which can be particularly important for those who are feeling isolated or lonely. Joining a fitness class, exercise group, or sports team can provide a sense of community and support, which can be beneficial for both physical and mental health.

It's important to note that exercise should not be used as the sole treatment for mental health conditions such as depression or anxiety. However, incorporating exercise into a larger treatment plan, including therapy or medication, can be an effective way to manage symptoms and improve overall mental well-being.

Improving Cognitive Function Through Exercise

Studies have shown that exercise can also have a positive impact on cognitive function, particularly in older adults. Regular exercise has been associated with improvements in attention, memory, and executive function, as well as a reduced risk of developing dementia.

The mechanisms behind the cognitive benefits of exercise are not fully understood, but researchers believe that exercise may increase blood flow to the brain, stimulate the growth of new brain cells, and promote the release of chemicals in the brain that support cognitive function.

There are many different types of exercise that may be beneficial for cognitive health, including aerobic exercise, strength training, and balance exercises. In particular, activities that involve both physical and cognitive demands, such as dancing or playing a sport, may be particularly effective.

It is important to note that the cognitive benefits of exercise are not limited to older adults. Studies have also found that children who are physically active tend to have better academic performance and cognitive function than their less active peers.

Overall, exercise appears to have numerous benefits for both physical and mental health, and should be incorporated into daily routines whenever possible.

Exercises for Mind and Body Connection (e.g., yoga, tai chi)

Mind and body exercises such as yoga, tai chi, and qigong are forms of exercise that aim to promote harmony between the mind and body. They involve slow, flowing movements, deep breathing, and meditation or mindfulness practices. These exercises are low-impact and gentle on the joints, making them suitable for people of all ages and fitness levels.

Yoga is a popular mind and body exercise that originated in ancient India. It combines physical postures, breathing techniques, and meditation or relaxation practices. Some of the physical benefits of yoga include increased flexibility, strength, and balance, as well as improved cardiovascular health. Yoga has also been found to reduce stress and anxiety, improve mood, and promote overall well-being.

Tai chi is a traditional Chinese mind and body exercise that involves slow, flowing movements and deep breathing. It is often described as "meditation in motion" and has been found to improve balance, flexibility, and strength, as well as reduce stress, anxiety, and depression. Tai chi has also been shown to improve cognitive function and reduce the risk of falls in older adults.

Qigong is another traditional Chinese mind and body exercise that involves gentle movements and deep breathing. It is often used to promote relaxation and reduce stress, as well as improve balance, flexibility, and overall physical health. Qigong has also been found to improve mental clarity and reduce symptoms of anxiety and depression.

Chapter 10

Frequently Asked Questions

How Often Should I Exercise?

The recommended frequency of exercise depends on the individual's age, fitness level, and overall health goals. The American Heart Association recommends at least 150 minutes of moderate-intensity aerobic exercise or 75 minutes of vigorous-intensity aerobic exercise per week, spread out over at least three days. It's also recommended to engage in strength training exercises at least two days per week.

For older adults, the Centers for Disease Control and Prevention recommends at least 150 minutes of moderate-intensity aerobic exercise per week, as well as balance training and muscle-strengthening activities at least two days per week.

It's important to note that any amount of physical activity is better than none, and even small amounts of exercise can provide health benefits. It's also important to listen to your body and adjust your exercise routine as necessary based on any health conditions or physical limitations.

What if I Have Limited Mobility?

If you have limited mobility, it's still important to find ways to stay active and get exercise. Even small amounts of activity can have benefits for your health and well-being.

There are many exercises and activities that can be modified or adapted to suit your needs and abilities. This may involve working with a physical therapist or other healthcare professional to develop a safe and effective exercise program.

Some exercises that may be suitable for those with limited mobility include chair exercises, resistance band exercises, water aerobics, and tai chi. It's important to start slowly and gradually increase the intensity and duration of your exercise as you become more comfortable and confident.

It's also important to listen to your body and avoid overexertion or pushing yourself too hard. Be sure to talk to your healthcare provider before starting any new exercise program, especially if you have any medical conditions or concerns.

Is it Safe to Exercise if I Have Other Health Conditions?

It is important to consult with a healthcare professional before starting an exercise program if you have any health conditions or concerns. In some cases, modifications or adjustments to your exercise routine may be necessary to ensure safety and prevent exacerbation of symptoms. Your healthcare provider can help determine what types of exercises and activities are appropriate for your individual needs and can also provide guidance on how to safely and effectively incorporate exercise into your routine. Additionally, it is important to listen to your body and modify your routine as needed based on how you feel during and after exercise.

What if I Have Never Exercised Before?

If you have never exercised before, it's important to start slowly and gradually increase the intensity and duration of your workouts. It's also a good idea to consult with a healthcare professional before beginning any new exercise program, especially if you have any pre-existing medical conditions or concerns.

Consider starting with low-impact exercises such as walking, swimming, or gentle yoga to build your endurance and improve your overall fitness level. You can also incorporate strength-training exercises using resistance bands or light weights to build muscle and improve balance.

Remember to listen to your body and stop or slow down if you experience pain or discomfort during exercise. It's also important to stay hydrated and fuel your body with nutritious foods to support your new exercise routine.

Don't be discouraged if you don't see immediate results. The benefits of exercise may take time to become apparent, but with consistency and dedication, you can improve your overall health and wellbeing.

Conclusion

The Benefits of Exercise for Frailty Syndrome

Frailty syndrome is a condition that affects many older adults and is characterized by decreased physical function, muscle weakness, and increased vulnerability to stressors such as illness or injury. Exercise can play a crucial role in managing and preventing frailty syndrome.

Some of the benefits of exercise for frailty syndrome include improved muscle strength, balance, coordination, and endurance. Exercise can also help to increase bone density and reduce the risk of falls and fractures.

Older adults with frailty syndrome may need to start with gentle exercises and gradually build up to more intense activities as their strength and endurance improve. Resistance training with light weights, resistance bands, or bodyweight exercises can help to improve muscle strength and function. Tai chi and yoga can also be beneficial for improving balance and coordination.

It's important for older adults with frailty syndrome to work with their healthcare provider and a qualified exercise professional to develop an exercise program that is safe and appropriate for their needs. Exercise should be tailored to the individual's abilities and should take into account any health conditions or medications that may affect their ability to exercise safely.

Here are some additional benefits of exercise for frailty syndrome:

1. Improved mobility and balance: Exercise can help to improve strength and balance, which can reduce the risk of falls and improve overall mobility.

2. Increased muscle mass: Resistance training and other forms of exercise can help to increase muscle mass, which can improve overall physical function.

3. Reduced risk of chronic diseases: Exercise can help to reduce the risk of chronic diseases such as heart disease, diabetes, and osteoporosis, which are more common in older adults with frailty syndrome.

4. Improved mental health: Exercise can also have positive effects on mental health, reducing symptoms of depression and anxiety and improving overall mood.

5. Increased social engagement: Participating in group exercise classes or activities can provide opportunities for social interaction and engagement, which is important for overall well-being.

It's important to note that exercise programs should be tailored to the individual's abilities and health status, and it's important to consult with a healthcare professional before starting a new exercise program.

Continuing Your Journey to Fitness and Independence.

Congratulations on taking the first steps towards a healthier and more active lifestyle! Remember that exercise is not a one-time thing, but a lifelong commitment to taking care of your body and mind. Here are some tips for continuing your journey to fitness and independence:

1. Set new goals: Once you have achieved your initial goals, it is important to set new ones to keep yourself motivated and challenged. These goals can be as

simple as increasing your daily step count or as ambitious as training for a marathon.

2. Try new activities: Don't be afraid to try new activities and mix up your routine. This will help prevent boredom and keep you engaged. Consider trying a new sport, dance class, or workout routine.

3. Incorporate strength training: As you age, it is important to maintain muscle mass and strength. Incorporating strength training exercises into your routine can help you achieve this. Talk to a trainer or physical therapist about safe and effective exercises.

4. Focus on balance and stability: As you age, your balance and stability may decrease, which can increase your risk of falls. Incorporating exercises that focus on balance and stability, such as

yoga or tai chi, can help prevent falls and improve your overall health.

5. Listen to your body: Pay attention to any aches or pains and adjust your exercise routine accordingly. If you are experiencing pain or discomfort, talk to a doctor or physical therapist to determine the best course of action.

Remember that exercise is just one piece of the puzzle when it comes to maintaining a healthy lifestyle. Be sure to also focus on a nutritious diet, staying hydrated, and getting enough rest and sleep. Congratulations again on taking the first steps towards a healthier you!